The Complete Guide To Kegel Exercises (Pelvic Floor)

A Complete Guide For Pelvic Wellness, Stronger, And A Healthier You

Aaron Mitchell Allen

Table of Contents

Introduction 4

CHAPTER ONE 8

    Kegel exercises 8

    The Benefits of Strong Pelvic Floor Muscles 12

    Kegels' Role in Core Stability and Health 15

CHAPTER TWO 19

    Understanding Your Pelvic Muscles 19

    The Structure and Function of Pelvic Floor Muscles 21

    Recognizing Core Muscles in Kegel Exercises 24

    Signs of Pelvic Floor Dysfunction and Weakness 26

CHAPTER THREE 29

    Proper Breathing Techniques for Effective Kegels 29

    Basic Kegel Exercises 31

    Step-by-Step Instructions for Performing Kegels 34

    Variations and Progressions to Challenge Your Muscles 37

CHAPTER FOUR 41

    Advanced Kegel Exercises 41

    Practical Kegel Exercises for Real-Life Use 43

    Kegels for Specific Conditions and Life Stages 46

    Kegel Exercises for Pregnancy and Postpartum Recovery 49

CHAPTER FIVE 51

    Managing Urinary Incontinence and Pelvic Organ Prolapse . 51

    Kegels for Sexual Health and Pleasure 53

    Pairing Kegels with Strength and Cardio Workouts 54

Creating a Balanced Workout for Pelvic Floor Health 57
CHAPTER SIX 61
    Tips for Long-Term Success 61
    Tackling Challenges And Staying Motivated 64
    Lifestyle and Diet for a Healthy Pelvic Floor 68
CHAPTER SEVEN 72
    Additional Therapies for Pelvic Health 72
    Conclusion 75
THE END 77

Introduction

Kegel exercises, named after Dr. Arnold Kegel who first introduced them, are a set of exercises designed to strengthen the pelvic floor muscles. The pelvic floor muscles play a crucial role in supporting the pelvic organs, controlling urinary and bowel functions, and maintaining sexual health. Despite their importance, these muscles often go unnoticed and can weaken over time due to factors like pregnancy, childbirth, aging, obesity, or a sedentary lifestyle.

Engaging in regular Kegel exercises can help improve and maintain the strength, endurance, and flexibility of the pelvic floor muscles. These exercises involve contracting and relaxing the muscles in a specific manner, targeting the deep muscles located between the pubic bone and tailbone. The beauty of Kegels is that they can be done discreetly, anytime and anywhere, without the need for any special equipment.

The benefits of strong pelvic floor muscles are numerous. They include improved bladder and bowel control, enhanced sexual function, prevention and management of pelvic organ prolapse, faster postpartum recovery, and relief from pelvic pain, and support during menopause. Kegel exercises empower individuals to take control of their pelvic floor wellness, promoting self-care, body awareness, and overall confidence.

Throughout this guide, we will delve deeper into the anatomy of the pelvic floor, the importance of these muscles in supporting and maintaining bodily functions, and how Kegel exercises can be incorporated into your daily routine. We will explore various techniques, progressions, and variations to help you get the most out of your Kegel exercises. Additionally, we will address common concerns, provide expert tips, and offer resources for further exploration.

By understanding the importance of Kegel exercises and embracing a regular practice, you can cultivate a strong and healthy pelvic floor, leading to improved well-being and a higher quality of life. Let's embark on this journey together and empower ourselves with the knowledge and tools to optimize our pelvic floor health.

CHAPTER ONE

Kegel exercises

Kegel exercises are a set of pelvic floor muscle exercises designed to strengthen and tone the muscles supporting the bladder, uterus, rectum, and small intestine. These exercises primarily target the pubococcygeus (PC) muscles, which play a vital role in controlling urinary flow and supporting pelvic organs.

Performing Kegels involves contracting and relaxing the pelvic floor muscles repetitively. They're often recommended for various reasons, including improving bladder control, preventing or alleviating urinary incontinence, enhancing sexual satisfaction, and aiding in postpartum recovery.

What's remarkable about Kegel exercises is their versatility and discreet nature. They can be done practically anywhere while sitting at a desk, watching TV, or even standing in line at the store without anyone noticing. This convenience allows individuals to incorporate them seamlessly into their daily routines.

Regular practice of Kegel exercises can lead to significant benefits. Strengthening these muscles may help in preventing leakage when coughing, sneezing, or laughing, which is particularly common in women after childbirth or during menopause. Additionally, stronger pelvic muscles can improve sexual function by enhancing sensations and improving control during intimacy.

It's important to perform Kegel exercises correctly to reap their full benefits. Identifying the right muscles is crucial; it involves contracting the muscles you'd use to stop the flow of urine or prevent passing gas. However, it's essential to note that Kegels should not be done while urinating as it can lead to incomplete emptying of the bladder and potential bladder infections.

Consistency is key with Kegel exercises. Like any muscle training, results take time, and it's essential to practice them regularly to notice improvements in pelvic strength and control. Consulting with a healthcare professional, especially for personalized guidance and ensuring proper technique, is advisable for those beginning Kegel exercises or experiencing specific pelvic health concerns.

The Benefits of Strong Pelvic Floor Muscles

Having strong pelvic floor muscles offers numerous benefits for both men and women. Here are some key advantages:

Improved bladder control: Strong pelvic floor muscles play a vital role in maintaining urinary continence. By strengthening these muscles, you can reduce the risk of urinary incontinence and have better control over urination, particularly during activities like coughing, sneezing, or lifting.

Enhanced bowel control: The pelvic floor muscles also contribute to bowel control. Strengthening them can help prevent fecal incontinence and promote regular bowel movements.

Support for pelvic organs: The pelvic floor provides support to the pelvic organs, including the bladder, uterus (in women), and rectum. Strong pelvic floor muscles help maintain proper organ positioning and reduce the risk of pelvic organ prolapse, a condition where the organs descend or bulge into the vaginal or rectal area.

Improved sexual function: Strong pelvic floor muscles can enhance sexual satisfaction for both men and women. These muscles play a role in sexual arousal, orgasm, and overall sexual well-being. Increased muscle tone and blood flow to the pelvic area can lead to improved sensations and better control during sexual activity.

Core stability and posture: The pelvic floor is an essential part of the core musculature. Strong pelvic floor muscles contribute to overall core stability, which supports good posture and spinal alignment. A stable core also helps in activities that require balance, stability, and strength.

Reduced back and pelvic pain: Strong pelvic floor muscles help provide support to the lower back and pelvis, which can reduce the risk of back pain and pelvic pain. This is especially beneficial for individuals with conditions like pelvic girdle pain or lower back pain.

Kegels' Role in Core Stability and Health

Kegel exercises are not just beneficial for the pelvic floor; they also contribute to core stability and overall health. Here's how:

Activation of deep core muscles: Kegel exercises involve activating the deep core muscles, including the transverse abdominis and multifidus muscles. These muscles, along with the pelvic floor, form the foundation of core stability.

Integrated core engagement: Incorporating Kegel exercises into your overall core training routine promotes integrated core engagement. By strengthening the pelvic floor along with other core muscles, such as the abdominals and back muscles, you enhance overall core stability and functional movement patterns.

Postural support: Strong pelvic floor muscles contribute to proper posture and alignment. They work in conjunction with other muscles of the core and back to support the spine, pelvis, and hips, reducing the risk of postural imbalances and associated pain.

Improved breathing mechanics: The pelvic floor muscles are connected to the diaphragm, the primary muscle involved in breathing. Proper engagement and coordination between the pelvic floor and diaphragm promote efficient breathing mechanics, aiding in relaxation, stress reduction, and overall well-being.

CHAPTER TWO

Understanding Your Pelvic Muscles

Understanding the anatomy of the pelvic floor is essential for effectively performing Kegel exercises. The pelvic floor is a group of muscles and tissues that form a supportive sling at the bottom of the pelvis. It consists of several key muscles:

Pubococcygeus (PC) muscles: These are the main muscles targeted in Kegel exercises. They stretch from the pubic bone at the front of the pelvis to the tailbone (coccyx) at the back. The PC muscles surround the openings of the urethra, vagina (in women), and rectum.

Bulbocavernosus muscles: These muscles lie on either side of the vaginal opening in women or the base of the penis in men. They are involved in sexual function and contribute to the strength of the pelvic floor.

Iliococcygeus muscles: Located towards the back of the pelvic floor, these muscles help support the pelvic organs and contribute to the overall stability of the pelvis.

Obturator internus muscles: These muscles wrap around the sides of the pelvis, assisting in pelvic floor function and stability.

Coccygeus muscles: These muscles extend from the tailbone to the ischial spine (part of the pelvis). They provide additional support to the pelvic floor and play a role in maintaining pelvic organ position.

The Structure and Function of Pelvic Floor Muscles

The pelvic floor muscles are a group of muscles that form a hammock-like structure at the bottom of the pelvis.

They play a crucial role in supporting the pelvic organs, controlling urinary and bowel functions, stabilizing the pelvis, and contributing to sexual function. Understanding the structure and function of these muscles is essential for effectively performing Kegel exercises.

The pelvic floor muscles consist of several layers, with each layer having specific functions:

Superficial layer: This layer includes the superficial transverse perineal muscles and the bulbospongiosus muscles.

These muscles help control the opening and closing of the urethra and vagina (in women) and assist in maintaining continence.

Intermediate layer: The intermediate layer consists of the external anal sphincter, which surrounds the anal canal and aids in controlling bowel movements.

Deep layer: The deep layer includes the pubococcygeus (PC) muscles, the puborectalis muscle, the iliococcygeus muscle, and the coccygeus muscle. These muscles provide support to the pelvic organs, assist in maintaining urinary and bowel continence, and contribute to pelvic stability.

Recognizing Core Muscles in Kegel Exercises

When performing Kegel exercises, it's important to identify and engage the key muscles of the pelvic floor. The primary muscle targeted in Kegels is the pubococcygeus (PC) muscle, which is part of the deep layer of the pelvic floor muscles. It stretches from the pubic bone at the front of the pelvis to the tailbone (coccyx) at the back.

To locate and engage the PC muscle, follow these steps:

Start by sitting or lying down in a comfortable position.

Imagine you're trying to stop the flow of urine midstream. Attempt to contract the muscles in that area without actually stopping the urine flow. These are the PC muscles.

Once you have identified the PC muscles, practice contracting and relaxing them without involving other muscles, such as the buttocks, thighs, or abdominal muscles.

Signs of Pelvic Floor Dysfunction and Weakness

Recognizing signs of pelvic floor dysfunction and weakness can help you understand if your pelvic floor muscles may require attention or targeted exercises like Kegels. Here are some common signs and symptoms to be aware of:

Urinary incontinence: If you experience involuntary urine leakage during activities such as coughing, sneezing, laughing, or exercising, it may indicate weakened pelvic floor muscles.

Bowel incontinence: Difficulty controlling bowel movements or experiencing unexpected fecal leakage can be a sign of pelvic floor weakness or dysfunction.

Pelvic organ prolapse: Symptoms of pelvic organ prolapse include a sensation of pressure or a bulge in the pelvic region, the feeling that the pelvic organs are dropping or protruding, or difficulty fully emptying the bladder or bowels.

Urinary urgency or frequency: Feeling a strong urge to urinate frequently, even when the bladder is not full, may indicate pelvic floor muscle dysfunction.

Pain in the pelvic region: Pelvic pain, including pain during intercourse (dyspareunia), pain in the genitals or perineum, or chronic pelvic pain, can be associated with pelvic floor dysfunction.

Lack of muscle tone or sensation: If you have difficulty sensing or engaging your pelvic floor muscles or if they feel weak or lax, it may indicate pelvic floor muscle weakness.

CHAPTER THREE

Proper Breathing Techniques for Effective Kegels

Proper breathing techniques are important during Kegel exercises as they help with muscle engagement, relaxation, and overall coordination. Here's a simple breathing technique to incorporate into your Kegel exercises:

Diaphragmatic breathing: Begin by finding a comfortable seated or lying position. Place one hand on your chest and the other hand on your abdomen, just below your ribcage.

Take a slow, deep breath in through your nose, allowing your abdomen to rise as you inhale. Focus on expanding your lower abdomen, feeling the breath fill your belly.

Exhale slowly through your mouth, allowing your abdomen to fall naturally as you breathe out.

Coordinate breath with muscle contractions: As you inhale, prepare for the muscle contraction by gently engaging your pelvic floor muscles. As you exhale, contract and lift your pelvic floor muscles, visualizing a gentle lift or squeeze.

Relax and release the pelvic floor muscles as you inhale again.

Repeat the cycle, coordinating your breath with the muscle contractions and releases.

Basic Kegel Exercises

Basic Kegel exercises provide a foundation for strengthening the pelvic floor muscles. Here's a step-by-step guide to get you started:

Find a comfortable position: Sit or lie down in a comfortable position. Make sure your body is relaxed, and your muscles are not overly tense.

Identify your pelvic floor muscles: Recall the sensation of stopping the flow of urine midstream or preventing the passage of gas. Contract the muscles in that area without actually urinating or passing gas. These are your pelvic floor muscles.

Contract and lift: Contract your pelvic floor muscles, lifting and squeezing them as strongly as you can without straining or causing discomfort. Hold the contraction for a few seconds, maintaining normal breathing throughout.

Relax and release: Slowly release the contraction, allowing your muscles to fully relax and lengthen. Take a moment to rest before repeating the exercise.

Repetitions and sets: Aim to perform 10-15 repetitions of the contractions in one session. Gradually increase the number of repetitions over time as your muscles become stronger.

Frequency: Initially, aim to do the exercises at least twice a day. As you progress, you can increase the frequency to three times a day or as recommended by a healthcare professional.

Step-by-Step Instructions for Performing Kegels

Performing Kegel exercises correctly is essential to effectively strengthen your pelvic floor muscles. Here's a step-by-step guide to help you perform Kegels:

Find a comfortable position: Choose a comfortable seated or lying position. Ensure your body is relaxed, and your muscles are not overly tense.

Identify your pelvic floor muscles: Recall the sensation of stopping the flow of urine midstream or preventing the passage of gas. Contract the muscles in that area without actually urinating or passing gas. These are your pelvic floor muscles.

Contract and lift: Gently contract your pelvic floor muscles, lifting and squeezing them as strongly as you can without straining or causing discomfort. Imagine pulling your pelvic floor muscles upward. Avoid tensing your abdomen, buttocks, or thigh muscles.

Hold the contraction: Hold the contraction for a few seconds, initially aiming for 3-5 seconds. Gradually increase the duration as your muscles become stronger. Maintain normal breathing throughout the contraction.

Relax and release: Slowly release the contraction, allowing your pelvic floor muscles to fully relax and lengthen. Take a moment to rest and breathe before repeating the exercise.

Repetitions and sets: Aim to perform 10-15 repetitions of the contractions in one session. Gradually increase the number of repetitions over time as your muscles become stronger. Start with one set of repetitions and gradually work your way up to three sets.

Frequency: Initially, aim to do the exercises at least twice a day. As you progress, you can increase the frequency to three times a day or as recommended by a healthcare professional.

Variations and Progressions to Challenge Your Muscles

Once you have mastered the basic Kegel exercises, you can introduce variations and progressions to further challenge and strengthen your pelvic floor muscles. Here are a few options to consider:

Longer contractions: Increase the duration of each contraction gradually. Instead of holding for a few seconds, aim to hold for 5-10 seconds or even longer as your muscles become stronger.

Quick contractions: Perform rapid, short contractions of the pelvic floor muscles. Contract and release the muscles quickly, aiming for a faster pace. This variation can help improve the dynamic strength and responsiveness of the pelvic floor.

Progressive resistance: Incorporate resistance by using Kegel exercise devices, such as weighted vaginal cones or resistance bands designed specifically for pelvic floor exercises. These devices provide added challenge and can enhance muscle strength and control.

Incorporating functional movements: Engage your pelvic floor muscles during functional movements, such as squats, lunges, or bridges. Practice contracting and lifting the pelvic floor while performing these exercises to promote integrated muscle engagement and functional strength.

CHAPTER FOUR

Advanced Kegel Exercises

As you advance in your Kegel exercises, you can incorporate more advanced techniques to further challenge your pelvic floor muscles. Here are some advanced Kegel exercises to consider:

Eccentric contractions: Instead of focusing solely on the contraction phase, emphasize the relaxation or lengthening phase of the muscle. Slowly and deliberately release the contraction, taking more time to relax the muscles than to contract them. This can improve muscle control and promote optimal muscle length-tension relationship.

Multi-dimensional contractions: Instead of only contracting the pelvic floor muscles in an upward direction, explore different directions of contraction. Try contracting and lifting the muscles forward, backward, and to the sides. This multidimensional approach can enhance overall muscle strength and coordination.

Integrated core exercises: Combine your Kegel exercises with other core exercises, such as planks, bird dogs, or

Pilates movements. Engage your pelvic floor muscles while performing these exercises to promote integrated core strength and stability.

Challenge your endurance: Increase the overall duration of your Kegel exercise sessions. Gradually work your way up to longer sessions, aiming for 10-15 minutes of continuous Kegel exercises. This can improve your pelvic floor muscle endurance.

Practical Kegel Exercises for Real-Life Use

Incorporating dynamic and functional movements into your Kegel exercises can help simulate real-world scenarios and improve muscle coordination and strength. Here are some examples of dynamic and functional Kegel exercises:

Squats with Kegel activation: Perform squats while actively engaging and lifting your pelvic floor muscles. As you lower into the squat, contract your pelvic floor, and maintain the contraction throughout the movement. This helps integrate pelvic floor activation into lower body exercises.

Lunges with Kegel activation: Perform lunges while engaging your pelvic floor muscles. As you step forward into a lunge, contract your pelvic floor, and maintain the contraction throughout the lunge. Alternate legs and continue to engage your pelvic floor with each repetition.

Bridge pose with Kegel activation: Lie on your back with your knees bent and feet flat on the floor. Lift your hips off the ground into a bridge pose while simultaneously engaging and lifting your pelvic floor muscles. Hold the bridge position and maintain the pelvic floor contraction. Lower your hips back down and repeat.

Kegels for Specific Conditions and Life Stages

Kegel exercises can be tailored to address specific conditions and life stages that impact pelvic floor health. Here are some examples:

Pregnancy and postpartum: Kegel exercises during pregnancy can help prepare the pelvic floor muscles for the physical demands of childbirth. After giving birth, Kegel exercises aid in postpartum recovery and help restore pelvic floor strength. Consult with a healthcare professional or pelvic floor specialist for specific guidance during pregnancy and postpartum.

Pelvic organ prolapse: If you have been diagnosed with pelvic organ prolapse, Kegel exercises can be part of a comprehensive treatment plan. Strengthening the pelvic floor muscles can help support the pelvic organs and potentially improve symptoms. However, the specific exercises and techniques should be determined in consultation with a healthcare professional.

Menopause: Hormonal changes during menopause can impact the pelvic floor muscles. Regular Kegel exercises can help maintain muscle tone, support bladder control, and improve overall pelvic floor health during this life stage.

Urinary incontinence: Kegel exercises are often recommended as a first-line treatment for stress urinary incontinence. By strengthening the pelvic floor muscles, you can improve bladder control and reduce leakage.

Kegel Exercises for Pregnancy and Postpartum Recovery

Kegel exercises are particularly beneficial during pregnancy and can aid in postpartum recovery. Here's how they can help:

Preparation for childbirth: Regularly practicing Kegel exercises during pregnancy can help strengthen the pelvic floor muscles, which can provide support during labor and delivery. Strong pelvic floor muscles may also help reduce the risk of perineal tears.

Postpartum recovery: After giving birth, Kegel exercises can aid in the recovery of the pelvic floor muscles, which may have been weakened or stretched during pregnancy and childbirth. Gradually incorporating Kegels into your postpartum routine can help restore strength and improve bladder control.

CHAPTER FIVE

Managing Urinary Incontinence and Pelvic Organ Prolapse

Kegel exercises are often recommended as a non-invasive approach for managing urinary incontinence and pelvic organ prolapse. Here's how they can help:

Urinary incontinence: Kegel exercises strengthen the pelvic floor muscles, which can help improve bladder control and reduce urinary leakage, particularly in cases of stress urinary incontinence. Consistent practice of Kegels can enhance the strength and endurance of the pelvic floor muscles, leading to improved bladder function.

Pelvic organ prolapse: Pelvic organ prolapse occurs when the pelvic organs descend or bulge into the vaginal or rectal area. Kegel exercises can help strengthen the pelvic floor muscles and provide support to the pelvic organs, potentially reducing the symptoms of pelvic organ prolapse. However, the specific exercises and techniques should be determined in consultation with a healthcare professional.

Kegels for Sexual Health and Pleasure

In addition to their functional benefits, Kegel exercises can also contribute to sexual health and pleasure. Here's how they can be beneficial:

Increased sensation and arousal: Strengthening the pelvic floor muscles through Kegel exercises can enhance blood flow to the pelvic region, leading to increased sensation and arousal during sexual activity. The improved muscle tone and control can contribute to greater sexual pleasure.

Enhanced orgasmic response: Well-toned pelvic floor muscles can lead to more intense and pleasurable orgasms. The ability to voluntarily contract and release the pelvic floor muscles can contribute to orgasmic control and intensify sexual experiences.

Pairing Kegels with Strength and Cardio Workouts

Combining Kegel exercises with strength training and cardiovascular exercises can create a well-rounded workout plan for pelvic floor health. Here's how you can integrate these components effectively:

Strength training: Incorporate Kegel exercises into your strength training routine by performing them during rest periods or between sets. For example, while doing a set of bicep curls, engage your pelvic floor muscles with a Kegel contraction. This helps to strengthen your pelvic floor muscles while working on other muscle groups.

Cardiovascular exercises: Engage your pelvic floor muscles during cardiovascular exercises such as walking, jogging, or using the elliptical machine. Focus on maintaining a consistent and rhythmic contraction of your pelvic floor muscles throughout your cardio workout.

Core exercises: Many core exercises, such as planks, bridges, and abdominal exercises, naturally engage the pelvic floor muscles. Incorporate Kegel exercises during these movements to enhance the activation of your pelvic floor muscles and strengthen your core as a whole.

Balance and flexibility exercises: Incorporate exercises that improve balance and flexibility, such as yoga or Pilates. During these exercises, focus on maintaining proper alignment and engaging your pelvic floor muscles to support stability and control.

Creating a Balanced Workout for Pelvic Floor Health

To design a well-rounded workout plan for pelvic floor health, consider the following tips:

Set specific goals: Determine your specific goals for pelvic floor health, such as improving bladder control, increasing muscle strength and endurance, or addressing specific pelvic floor conditions. Tailor your workout plan to align with these goals.

Start with a warm-up: Begin each workout session with a warm-up that includes gentle movements, dynamic stretches, and activation exercises for the whole body, including the pelvic floor muscles.

Incorporate Kegel exercises: Dedicate specific time within your workout routine for focused Kegel exercises. Perform them with proper technique, gradually increasing intensity, duration, and variations as your pelvic floor muscles become stronger.

Include strength training: Integrate strength training exercises that target major muscle groups while incorporating Kegel exercises. This helps to promote overall muscle strength and stability, which supports the pelvic floor.

Include cardiovascular exercises: Include cardiovascular exercises like walking, running, cycling, or swimming in your routine. Engage your pelvic floor muscles while maintaining proper breathing and form throughout the exercises.

Emphasize core exercises: Prioritize exercises that target the core muscles, such as planks, bridges, and Pilates movements. These exercises naturally engage the pelvic floor muscles and promote overall core strength.

Allow for rest and recovery: Ensure that you include rest days and recovery periods in your workout plan. Resting allows your muscles, including the pelvic floor muscles, to recover and adapt to the exercise stimulus.

CHAPTER SIX

Tips for Long-Term Success

To maintain consistency and make progress with your pelvic floor workout plan, consider the following tips:

Set a regular schedule: Establish a consistent schedule for your workouts, including dedicated time for Kegel exercises. This helps to build a routine and makes it easier to stick to your plan.

Set reminders: Use reminders, alarms, or calendar notifications to prompt and remind you to do your pelvic floor exercises. This can help you stay on track and avoid skipping sessions.

Track your progress: Keep a record of your workouts and track your progress over time. Note the duration, intensity, and variations of your exercises. This helps you stay motivated and allows you to monitor your improvement.

Gradually increase intensity: As your pelvic floor muscles become stronger, gradually increase the intensity, duration, and resistance of your exercises. This progressive overload ensures continued improvement and challenges your muscles.

Seek guidance when needed: If you have specific pelvic floor concerns or conditions, consider seeking guidance from a healthcare professional or pelvic floor specialist. They can provide personalized recommendations, modifications, and support to help you achieve your goals.

Listen to your body: Pay attention to your body's signals during exercises. If you experience pain, discomfort, or any unusual symptoms, adjust your technique or consult with a healthcare professional.

Stay motivated: Find ways to stay motivated and make your workouts enjoyable. This can include listening to music, exercising with a friend, joining a class, or incorporating other activities you enjoy alongside your pelvic floor exercises.

Tackling Challenges And Staying Motivated

Challenges and hurdles are normal on any wellness journey. Here are some strategies to overcome common challenges and stay motivated:

Consistency is key: Make a commitment to consistency in your pelvic floor exercises. Establish a routine and stick to it, even on days when motivation is low. Consistent effort over time leads to progress and results.

Find an accountability partner: Partner up with a friend, family member, or workout buddy who shares similar goals. Keep each other accountable, provide support, and motivate one another to stay on track.

Mix it up: Avoid getting bored or plateauing by incorporating variety into your exercises. Explore different Kegel variations, try new fitness classes, or engage in activities that challenge and engage your pelvic floor muscles in different ways.

Seek professional guidance: If you encounter difficulties or have specific concerns, consult with a healthcare professional or pelvic floor specialist. They can provide guidance, modify exercises to suit your needs, and address any challenges you may face.

Focus on the benefits: Remind yourself of the numerous benefits of pelvic floor health, such as improved bladder control, enhanced sexual satisfaction, and better overall quality of life. Keep these benefits in mind when motivation wanes.

Reward yourself: Set up a reward system for reaching specific milestones or consistently sticking to your exercise routine. Treat yourself to something you enjoy, such as a massage, a new workout outfit, or a relaxing activity.

Stay educated and inspired: Continuously educate yourself about pelvic floor health and stay inspired through books, podcasts, online resources, or workshops. Learning more about the topic and hearing success stories can help you stay motivated.

Lifestyle and Diet for a Healthy Pelvic Floor

In addition to exercise and holistic approaches, nutrition and lifestyle factors play a crucial role in supporting optimal pelvic floor function. Here are some considerations:

Hydration: Drinking an adequate amount of water is important for overall health and can contribute to optimal pelvic floor function. Aim to stay hydrated by consuming enough fluids throughout the day.

Fiber-rich diet: A diet high in fiber promotes regular bowel movements and helps prevent constipation, which can strain the pelvic floor muscles. Include fiber-rich foods such as fruits, vegetables, whole grains, and legumes in your diet.

Healthy weight management: Maintaining a healthy weight is important for pelvic floor health. Excess weight can put additional strain on the pelvic floor muscles. Focus on adopting a balanced and nutritious diet and engaging in regular physical activity to support a healthy weight.

Avoiding constipation: Chronic constipation can lead to straining during bowel movements, which can negatively impact the pelvic floor. Ensure you have a diet rich in fiber, drink plenty of water, and establish regular bowel habits to prevent constipation.

Proper lifting techniques: When lifting heavy objects, it's important to use proper technique to avoid placing excessive strain on the pelvic floor muscles. Lift with your legs, keep your back straight, and engage your core muscles to provide support.

Posture and body mechanics: Maintaining good posture and body mechanics throughout daily activities can help minimize stress and strain on the pelvic floor. Be mindful of your posture when sitting, standing, and performing various movements.

CHAPTER SEVEN

Additional Therapies for Pelvic Health

In addition to Kegel exercises and lifestyle factors, there are various therapeutic techniques and modalities that can support pelvic health. These may be particularly beneficial when working with a healthcare professional or pelvic floor specialist. Here are a few examples:

Manual therapy: Hands-on techniques provided by a pelvic floor physical therapist, such as myofascial release or trigger point therapy, can help release tension and optimize muscle function in the pelvic floor.

Biofeedback: Biofeedback is a technique that provides real-time information about muscle activity. It can help you better understand and gain control over your pelvic floor muscles by providing visual or auditory cues.

Electrical stimulation: Electrical stimulation involves using mild electrical currents to stimulate and strengthen the pelvic floor muscles. This technique is often used under the guidance of a healthcare professional.

Pelvic floor physical therapy: Pelvic floor physical therapy is a specialized form of therapy that focuses on assessing and treating pelvic floor dysfunction. A pelvic floor physical therapist can provide personalized guidance, education, and exercises tailored to your specific needs.

Relaxation techniques: Practicing relaxation techniques such as deep breathing, meditation, or mindfulness can help reduce tension and promote relaxation in the pelvic floor muscles.

Conclusion

Embracing a stronger and healthier pelvic floor is an important aspect of overall well-being. By incorporating Kegel exercises, holistic approaches, and considering nutrition and lifestyle factors, you can support optimal pelvic floor function and improve your quality of life.

Remember that pelvic floor health is a journey, and progress may take time. It's important to be patient, listen to your body, and seek guidance from healthcare professionals or pelvic floor specialists when needed. With dedication, consistency, and a holistic approach, you can embrace a stronger and healthier pelvic floor, supporting your overall wellness and enjoying the benefits of improved bladder control, enhanced sexual health, and greater confidence in your daily life.

THE END

www.ingramcontent.com/pod-product-compliance
Lightning Source LLC
Chambersburg PA
CBHW071841210526
45479CB00001B/238